I0837384

THE ESSENTIAL GUIDE TO CANNABIS

DOSAGES, COOKING, PETS, MEDICAL APPLICATIONS AND MORE

Deana E Jones

FOUNDER of

Springville Sun Organics CBD

Table of Contents

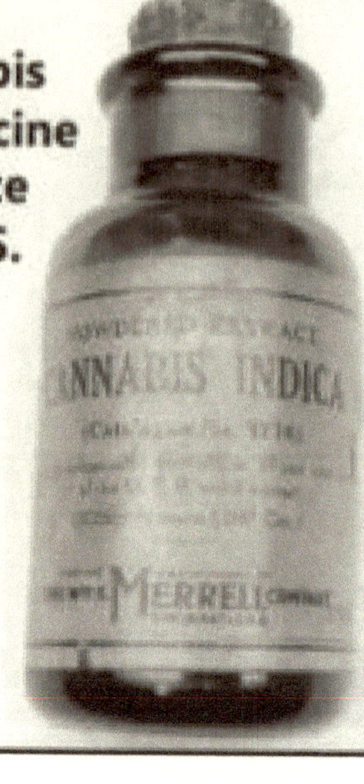

From 1850 to 1937, cannabis was used as the prime medicine for more than 100 separate illnesses or diseases in U.S. Pharmacopoeia.

Chapter 1

History of Human Use

Cannabis Sativa is from the Cannabaceae family of flowering plants. It has a long history of cultivation for its physical attributes, its medicinal benefits and recreational purposes.

Cannabis is commonly called marijuana, weed, grass, or pot in popular culture. It is related to, but different than, cannabis cultivated for industrial purposes, which is called hemp.

Industrial hemp is grown primarily for the seeds, oils, stalks, and fibers and contains fewer *cannabinoids* (which we will discuss later) than medicinal cannabis. Cannabis (marijuana) contains high levels of chemical compounds called cannabinoids, which lead to its many medical benefits and recreational purposes.

Cannabis was cultivated by humans as early as 4,000 B.C. Archaeologists have uncovered the first evidence of use in China, which used the plant for fibers, medicine and food.

However, there is some indication of use for the psychoactive experience. The plant soon traveled along trade routes from China to India, where it became an integral aspect of cultural and religious traditions. Around 450 B.C., cannabis entered into Europe, and Europeans used the plants for its fibers and possibly for ceremonial traditions. In the 19th century, Western medicine adopted cannabis as a therapeutic agent. After a period of prohibition in North America and Europe, some countries and regions have reintroduced cannabis as medicine and for recreational purposes.

Cannabis Strains

The origins of all strains today come from the Asiatic continent. There is some indication indica evolved into a sub variation on the Indian subcontinent. Sativa developed closer to the equator. Cannabis nomenclature remains unstable. The popular distinction between indica and sativa strains of cannabis continues, but the genetic distinction is arguable.

There is proven genetic variation, but it may not be accurately represented by the popular strains, nor on dispensary labels.

The continued differentiation between the two strains in popular culture, while unproven, is persistent. The differences are complicated by the hybridization between strains, and regional variations. Popular strains at dispensaries may have all or none of the characteristics described below:

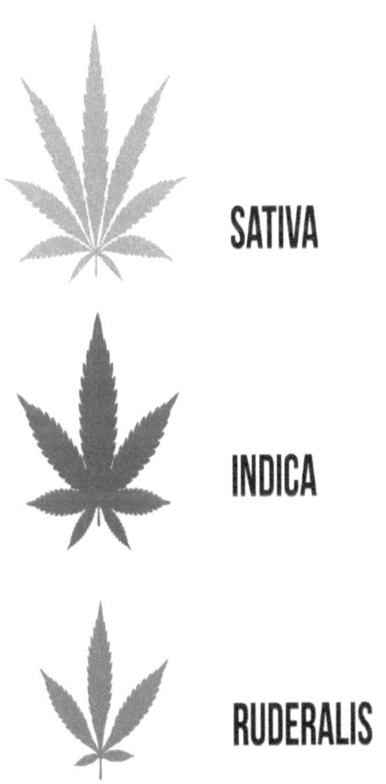

CANNABIS SATIVA:

Experience: creative, euphoric, uplifting, energizing.

Potential therapeutic values: mood lifting (anxiety, depression), day-time use.

Physical appearance: Grows between 5 to 18 ft. tall, thinly leaved, few branches.

Popular strains: Durban, Poison, Jack Herer, Haze.

CANNABIS INDICA:

Experience: sedative, relaxing, commonly referred to as "couch lock"

Potential therapeutic values: *sedation, pain relief, reduces nausea, improves appetite, night- time use.*

Physical Appearance: *Grows 2-4 ft. tall, broad leaved, compact leaves and branches, bushy appearance, wider flowers.*

Popular strains: *Bubba Kush, Blueberry, Blue Cheese.*

CANNABIS RUDERALIS:

Experience: *Poorly understood, less powerful than indica or sativa.*

Potential therapeutic values: *Low THC, less understood*

Physical Appearance: *Grows under 2 ft. tall, unbranched, autoflowering, rare.*

Popular strains: *due to low THC content it is rarely used outside of hybrid combinations.*

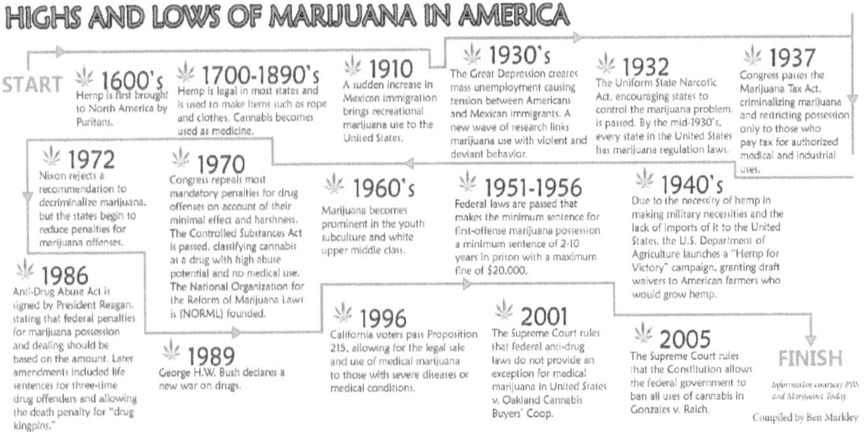

Figure 1 - Highs and Lows of Marijuana in the U.S.

One hundred years ago, the federal government was not overly concerned with marijuana, the common name for the Cannabis sativa L. plant. Initially spelled "marihuana," it was also known as hemp, Mary Jane, Mary Warner, and by variety of other terms. Most Americans seemed unaware of its presence, let alone its exploitation as a drug.

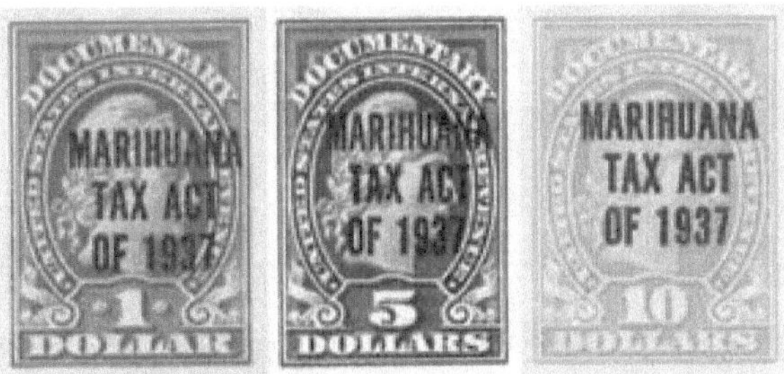

Marihuana Tax Act of 1937 stamp required for legal import and export of the drug.

By the 1930s, several state governments and other countries had banned the drug. The U.S. government hesitated, in part because therapeutic uses of Cannabis were still being explored and American industry profited from commercial applications of hemp fiber, seeds and oil.

Marijuana was not classed as a major drug-unlike opium and heroin, which were prohibited under the Harrison Narcotics Tax Act of 1914 and subsequent restrictive legislation. As the political climate changed, Federal Bureau of Narcotics Commissioner Harry Anslinger became a powerful anti-marijuana voice. His campaign against Cannabis led to the passage of the Marihuana Tax Act of 1937, under which the importation, cultivation, possession and/or distribution of marijuana were regulated.

Among the act's provisions was one requiring the importers to register and pay an annual tax of $24. A Marihuana Tax Act stamp, affixed to each original order form and marked by the revenue collector, insured that proper payments were made. The custom's collector held custody of imported marijuana at the port of entry until required documents were received, with similar regulations governing marijuana exports. Shipments were subject to searches, seizures and forfeitures if any provisions of the law were not met. Violation of the act resulted in a fine of not more than $2,000 and/or imprisonment for up to five years.

In principle, the Marihuana Tax Act of 1937 stopped only the use of the plant as a recreational drug. In practice, though, industrial hemp was caught up in anti-dope legislation, making hemp importation and commercial production in this country less economical. Scientific research and medical testing of marijuana also virtually disappeared. By 1970, marijuana was classified and restricted on par with narcotics and new, tighter laws were enacted. Changes have occurred over the last 40 years. As of January 2012, 16 states and the District of Columbia have legalized marijuana for medical purposes, though this is still not permitted under federal regulations.

Just prior to the passage of the Marihuana Tax Act of 1937, the Customs Agency Service compiled a Narcotics Manual that reported: "Marihuana may be cultivated or grown wild in almost any locality. Inasmuch as this drug is so readily obtained in the United States, it is not believed to be the subject of much organized smuggling from other countries." Today, however, marijuana trafficking is a major concern of CBP, Immigration and Customs Enforcement and the Drug Enforcement Administration. Well over 3 million pounds of "pot" were confiscated at our borders in 2011, making an impact on this multibillion-dollar illegal enterprise.

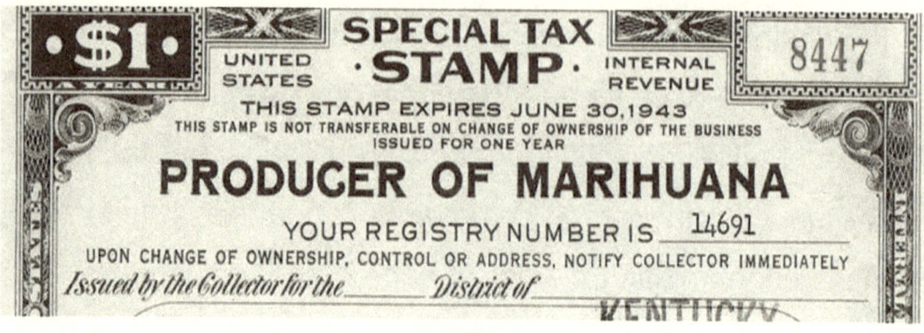

Figure 2 - Marijuana Tax Stamp

Chapter 2

Consumption Methods

SMOKING

Finely ground cannabis flowers or concentrates such as shatter, wax, oils and hash can be used
Smoking requires incineration by flame in a pipe, bong, bubbler, one-hitter, joint or blunt. Smoking is still the most common and preferred option among cannabis users. There is continued debate about the health effects of smoking cannabis, and its value as a therapeutic option is in question.
<ul><li>Effects are short term, usually between 2 to 6 hours.</li><li>Effects are quick in onset, usually within 5 to 15 minutes.</li><li>Effects are not as potent as an edible.</li><li>Used for the treatment of health issues which require quick, targeted therapy including mood disorders (anxiety, depression), acute pain and inflammation, insomnia.</li></ul>

VAPORIZING

Concentrates or raw flower is used, heated through convection or induction, with a tabletop, dab rig, or handheld device.
Commonly called vaping, is a relatively new and popular method of consumption. Instead of incineration, it vaporizes the oily cannabinoids through induction and convection heat sources. It does not combust organic material and is therefore assumed to be healthier than smoking raw flower. Researchers

have not yet proven the accuracy of this assumption.
• Effects are short term, usually between 2 and 6 hours. • Effects are quick in onset, usually within 5 to 15 minutes. • Effects are not as potent as an edible. • Used for the treatment of health issues which require quick, targeted therapy including mood disorders (anxiety and depression), acute pain and inflammation, insomnia.

EDIBLE

Baked goods, cooking oils, candles, ice creams, savory main dishes, etc., are used
Edible cannabis is the infusions of the raw cannabis into oils, butters and tinctures. The infusion is then incorporated into foodstuffs. They are highly adaptable to personal taste and dietary restrictions. Due to their potency and slow onset, they are also the cause of the majority of marijuana overdoses, also known as acute marijuana intoxication.
• Effects are long lasting, usually between 6 to 8 hours. • Effects are slow on onset, as long as 2 or more hours after ingestion. • Usually with high levels of THC, 100 mg or more. • Used for the treatment of chronic illness, which requires long lasting treatment such as: nausea and vomiting, pain, and insomnia.

TOPICAL

Creams, salves, oils and balms are used
Topical applications are the only cannabis products which do not trigger a psychoactive reaction, no matter the THC content. The cannabinoids do not

enter the bloodstream. Instead, the cannabinoids permeate only the skin's surface to influence the CB2 receptions concentrated in the epidermis. Despite the increasing popularity of topical cannabis applications, there is conflicting research about its medicinal value.

- Effects are non-psychoactive.
- Products often contain CBD, and low levels of THC.

- Used for the treatment of skin issues and joint inflammation, including pain associated with arthritis, sore joints and muscles, psoriasis, eczema and other skin irritations.

Cannabis Products

With the improved access to legal cannabis, there is now a wide variety of products and brands available. The more refined a cannabis product, the higher the potency. Concentrates use heat, time, and/or pressure to extract the valuable cannabinoids and terpenes. Often, many of the lesser, more sensitive compounds are lost during the high-heat processing of an extraction.

RAW FLOWER

The cured raw flower of the cannabis plant is obtained in a full flower format or fine grind. It contains all the natural cannabinoids and terpenes and is often referred to as the 'whole plant' preparation.

- Suitable for smoking, vaping, and make at home edibles.

- Potencies vary up to approximately 30% THC.

- The most common format of cannabis.

CONCENTRATES

A cannabis concentrate is the concentration of the raw flower into a higher potency product. Concentrates are often preferred for chronic illness, due to their higher potency and ease of use.

- Suitable for smoking, vaping, dabbing edibles.

- Typically contains 30 to 99% cannabinoid content.

- Produced via: solvent extraction (butane, ethanol, CO2), rosin extraction (heat and pressure), agitation (crystal collection for hash).

- Common concentrates: alcohol tincture, shatter, hash, waxsugar, phoenix tears, butter, butane honey oil.

Chapter 3

History of Medical Marijuana

What is medical marijuana or medical cannabis?

Medical marijuana is the medical use of the *Cannabis sativa* or *Cannabis indica* plant to relieve symptoms or treat diseases and conditions. The *Cannabis* plant was used medically for centuries around the world until the early 1900s. Medical marijuana facts can be difficult to find because strong opinions exist, both pros and cons.

What are THC and CBD?

THC or tetrahydrocannabinolis the psychoactive compound in marijuana. It is responsible for the "high" people feel. There are two man-made drugs
called dronabinol (Marinol) and nabilone (Cesamet) that are synthetic forms of THC. They are FDA-approved to prevent nausea and vomiting in people receiving chemotherapy.

CBD or cannabidiol is another compound in marijuana that is not psychoactive. CBD is thought to be responsible for the majority of the medical benefits.

Epidiolex is a CBD oil extract that is undergoing clinical trials for epilepsy.

THC: CBD: Nabiximols (Sativex) is a specific plant extract with an equal ratio of THC:CBD. It is approved as a drug in the UK and elsewhere in Europe for the treatment of multiple sclerosis, spasticity, neuropathic pain, overactive bladder and other indications.

Medical marijuana products are available with a huge range of THC and CBD concentrations. Expert opinion states that 10mg of THC should be considered "one serving" and a person new to medical marijuana should inhale or consume no more until they know their individual response.

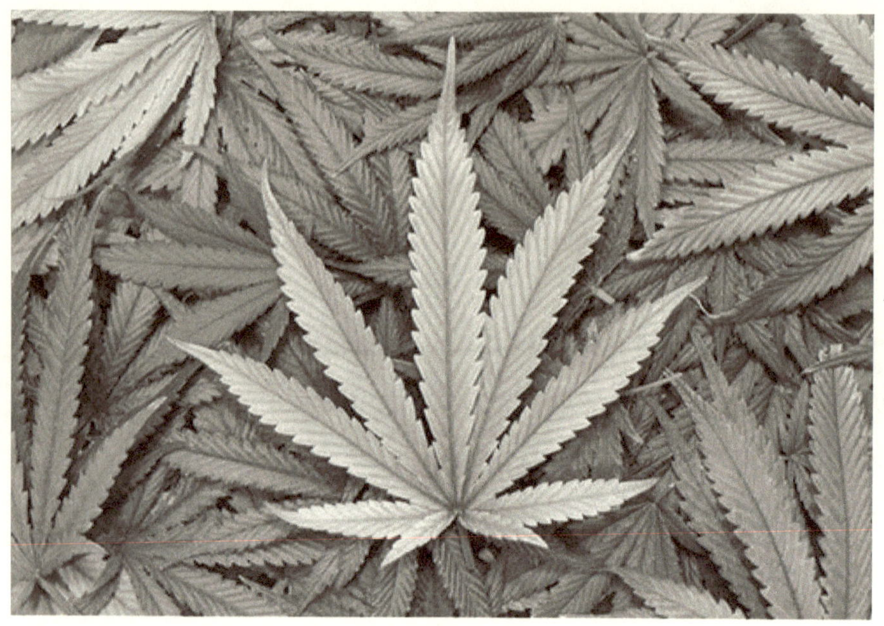

Legislation regarding cannabis continues to this day to fluctuate, what may be legal today could be deemed illegal tomorrow.

As of this writing, the **Hemp Farming Act** of 2018 was a proposed law to remove hemp (defined as cannabis with less than 0.3% THC) from Schedule I controlled substances and making it an ordinary agricultural commodity. Its provisions were incorporated in the 2018 United States farm bill that became law on December 20, 2018.

This farm bill taking effect opened up a booming industry of CBD products across the nation, and today you can easily find CBD products on every corner, including gas stations. CBD is discussed more thoroughly in this book, in Chapter 4. There are caveats with CBD however, such as THC content contained in the products being legal and if there is any CBD in the products and if so, how much? The booming CBD industry of today has allowed a lot of snake oil salesmen to profit due to the fact that there are still many unanswered questions and the lack of education of the public on these matters.

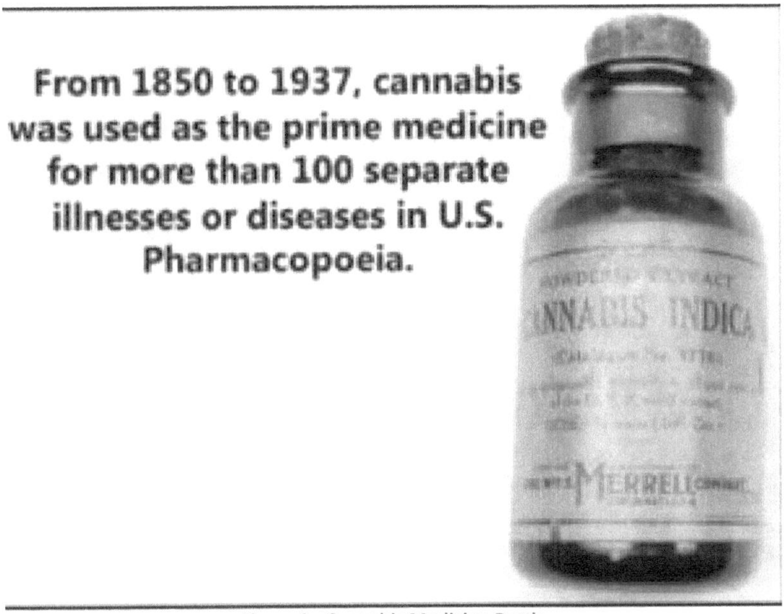

From 1850 to 1937, cannabis was used as the prime medicine for more than 100 separate illnesses or diseases in U.S. Pharmacopoeia.

Figure 3 - Cannabis Medicine Bottle

Medical Applications

Medical Marijuana is an all-natural alternative therapy, popular in Eastern and Western medical traditions. Legally available through a medical marijuana card, or certified prescription in many places in North America and Europe. Individual regulations and accessibility will vary, check local laws for details. Under physician care, patients often self-direct dosing protocols including marijuana product, the method of ingestions, dose, and timing. Medical marijuana may be appropriate for chronic or acute health concerns. Marijuana has a high safety profile in most circumstances, even with long term use.

Approved medical conditions and diseases are:

ADD/ADHD	AIDS/HIV
Alzheimer's Disease	Amyotrophic lateral sclerosis (ALS)
Anorexia	Anxiety
Arnold Chiari malformation	Arthritis
Autism	Auto Accident(s)
Back and Neck Problems	Brain Injury
Cachexia	Cancer
Causalgia	Cerebral palsy
Cervical dystonia	Chronic inflammatory demyelinating
Chronic nausea	Chronic nervous system disorders
Chronic pain	Chronic pancreatitis
Chronic traumatic encephalopathy	Colitis
Complex regional pain syndrome	Crohn's disease
Cystic fibrosis	Debilitating epilepsy
Depression	Dystonia
Eating disorders	Ehlers-Danlos syndrome
Epilepsy or other seizure disorders	Fibromyalgia
Fibrous dysplasia	Gastrointestinal disorders
Glaucoma	Hepatitis C

HIV/Aids	Huntington's Disease
Hydromyelia	Inflammatory Bowel Disease (IBD)
Irreversable Spinal Cord Injury	Irritable Bowel Syndrome
Kidney Failure/Dialysis	Lupus
Migraine	Mitchondrial disease
Multiple Sclerosis	Muscle Spasms
Muscular Dystrophy	Myasthenia Gravis
Myoclonus	Nail-patella syndrome
Nausea	Neurofibromatosis
Neuropathies	Parkinson's Disease
Polyneuropathy	Postlaminectomy syndrome
Post-concussion syndrome	Post-Traumatic Stress Disorder
Reflex sympathetic dystrophy (RSD)	Rheumatoid Arthritis
Severe Arthritis	Sexual Dysfunction
Sickle Cell Anemia	Sjogren's syndrome
Sleep disorders	Spinal cord damage
Spinal cord injury/disease	Spinal stenosis
Spinocerebellar ataxia (SCA)	Syringomyelia
Tarlov cysts	Terminal illness
Tourettes's syndrome	Traumatic brain injury
Ulcerative colitis	~~~~~

Of course, metabolism, body size, and genetics may all influence how quickly and how strongly medical marijuana takes effect. Muscle mass and fat tissue may affect tolerance. There is evidence suggesting mean and women experience medical marijuana differently. Women may react more strongly to THC, as they have fewer THC mediating receptors. Sex hormones also influence the strength of THC. Seniors are generally more sensitive to THC than younger adults. With frequent use over prolonged periods, tolerance to THC builds. The CB1 receptors become desensitized to the constant flood of THC. Taking time off from continuous THC exposure can resolve this issue. Every strain and cannabis product contain different blends of cannabinoids. Strains and products with a higher percentage of THC produce more powerful effects. The addition of CBD may reduce the effects of THC. Inhaling marijuana generally provides immediate, but short-term relief. Edibles and sublingual delivery take longer to go into effect but have longer lasting relief.

The United States now has a medical marijuana card program. The figure on the following page shows the states that currently offer this program.

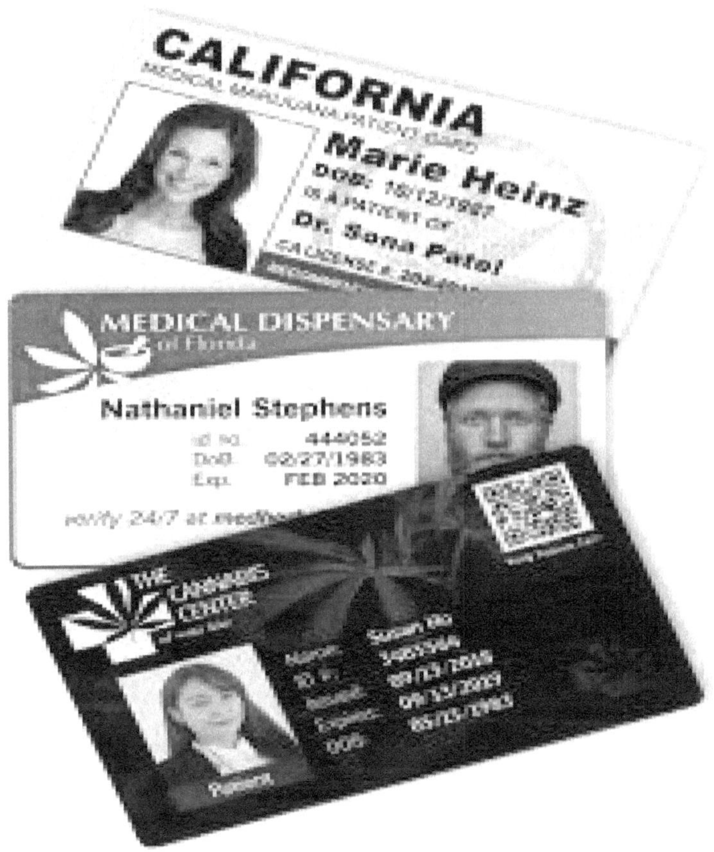

Figure 4 - Medical Marijuana Cards

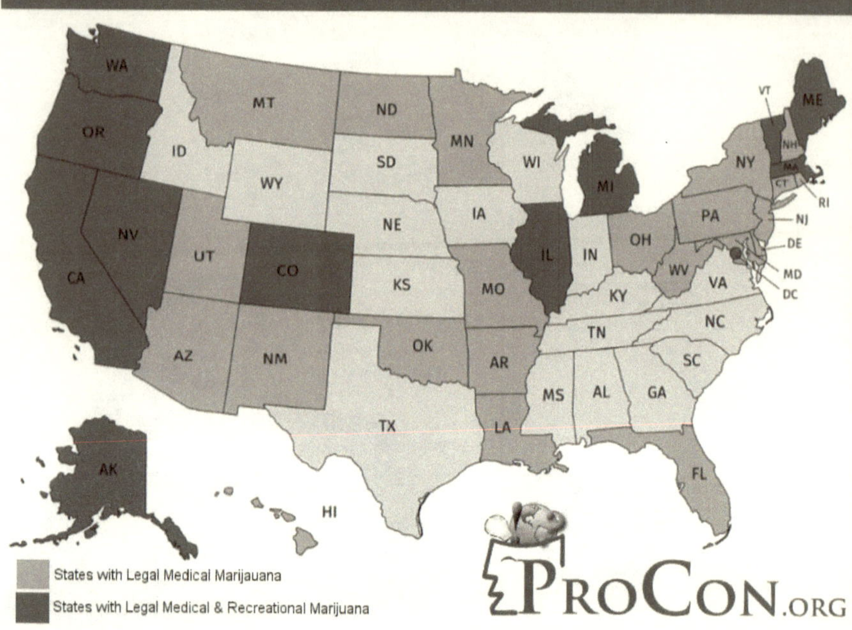

Figure 5 - Legal Medical Marijuana States

Known Risks and Adverse Side Effects

The popular claim that there are no deaths directly associated with cannabis are technically true but ignores the many adverse side effects and long-term risk factors associated with cannabis use. The risk and adverse side effects of cannabis are almost exclusively related to the only psychoactive cannabinoid: THC. Cannabidiol (CBD) continues to prove safe for human consumption even in large doses. Due to the non-psychoactive nature of all other cannabinoids, their risk profile is also largely assumed to be relatively safe.

ADVERSE SIDE EFFECTS	SHORT TERM RISKS	LONG TERM RISKS
The immediate and short -term adverse side effects of cannabis use, are typically associated with THC. They may include: - Paranoia - Anxiety - Impaired short- term memory - Altered judgment and increased risk taking - Sedation	The short- term health risks associated with cannabis use, typically are not associated with the cannabinoid profile. Usually the short- term health risks are associated with method of consumption, mainly smoking. Short term risks include: - Increased risk for the development of bronchitis - Chronic	The long -term risks associated with cannabis use are low but may prove severe. Long term health risks include: - Increased risk for one subtype of testicular cancer. - Prenatal use of cannabis may increase risk of

- Acute marijuana intoxication In some rare cases, CBD may cause the following adverse side effects: - Diarrhea - Tiredness - Changes in appetite and weight	cough, and increased phlegm production - Increased risk of death and injury associated with risk taking and driving impairment.	cancer in the offspring - Increased risk of developing schizophrenia and other psychosis - Regular use may increase suicidal thoughts with depression - Regular use may increase symptoms of bipolar disorder - Increased risk for developing social anxiety disorder - Regular use associated with higher risk for cannabis use disorder (dependency)

CAUTION! Synthetic Cannabinoids

Synthetic cannabinoids are chemical compounds produced in a laboratory they are not sourced from natural sources. Illicit synthetic cannabinoids are untested and used illegally around the world as an intoxicant. More than 125 recorded illicit synthetic cannabinoids exist globally. Examples are **K2 and Spice**. There is a higher risk of addiction than natural cannabinoids and higher risk of serious side effects than natural cannabinoids. There is NO known medicinal benefits from these synthetic products, and they are untested and unregulated.

Pharmaceutical synthetic cannabinoids are used globally for specific approved conditions and are developed to mimic the effects of phytocannabinoids in cannabis, but they also avoid regulatory issues. Examples include drobinol and nabilone both which target nausea and vomiting associated with chemotherapy. Drobinal is also approved for use for the treatment of HIV/AIDS induced anorexia.

Chapter 4

CBD

Once the Farm Bill Act of 2018 was signed into law, the CBD/Hemp Oil industry took the market by storm! Little bottles of CBD oil flooded into gas stations, multi-level marketing companies, online companies and a few scattered brick and mortar stores. The craze left several confusing voids in the new industry including absent or little regulation, misunderstanding of what CBD is and the purpose of it, as well as the mistaken belief that CBD would "produce the high that a person experiences from smoking marijuana." There remains strong opposition from Christian groups yet surprisingly, many 'members of the congregation' are consuming CBD behind closed doors due to the presently lingering stigma of marijuana from decades earlier, along with fear of backlash.

When I started my CBD company, the struggle was real! CBD was a hot item and I assumed that I would do very well, however I was sadly mistaken. I had no idea of the hoops I would have to jump through just to be facing a brick wall in the end. Advertising restrictions on just about every platform almost choked the life out of my little struggling company. It was nearly impossible to get the word out about my new company and the benefits of CBD. I was chased out of the door of several businesses that I wanted to place my products in, with the owners yelling after me that I was 'selling the work of the devil' and that I was 'just a drug addict trying to make a score.' Yes, this actually happened to me! So much misinformation, lack of education, and in my opinion, just plain ignorance.

I finally realized that I would have to start education people any way I could, to those who would at least listen. In some ways, I couldn't really blame the naysayers, because I myself was more than a little hesitant at first to try CBD oil for some back issues that I had. The old stigmas remain, and there are some people that have actually changed their previous favorable opinion of my reputation, to a not so good one once they found out that I entered the cannabis business.

However, I stood my ground always having believed that natural healing is the best avenue of healing and CBD is one, if not the number one option to get there.

It is now known that Baby Boomers are in fact the largest group of consumers of CBD oil. The reasons for this are because CBD oil is known to relieve pain and inflammation, two big issues that those in their later years suffer the most from.

For many people experiencing chronic pain, cannabidiol (CBD) oil has steadily gained popularity as a natural approach to pain relief. A compound found in the marijuana plant, cannabidiol is sometimes touted as an alternative to pain medication in the treatment of common conditions like arthritis and back pain.

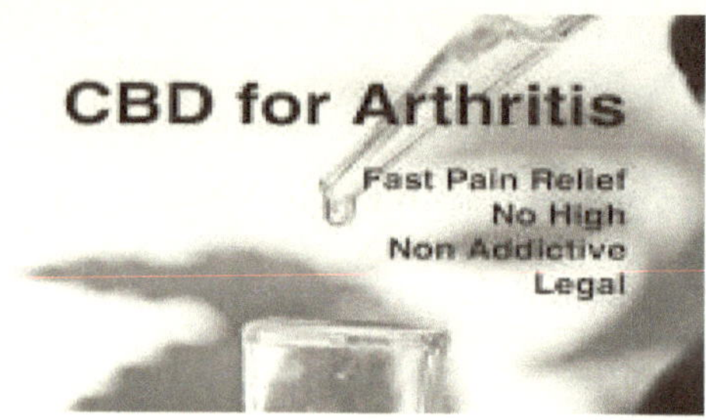

Figure 6 - CBD Oil

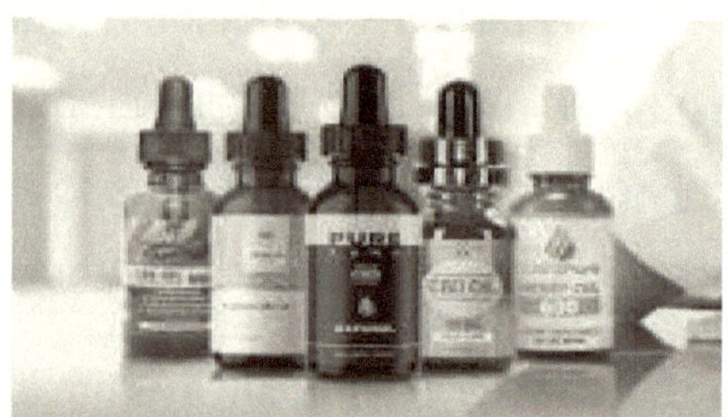

CBD stands for cannabidiol. It is the second most prevalent of the active ingredients of cannabis (marijuana). While CBD is an essential component of medical marijuana, it is derived directly from the hemp plant, which is a cousin of the marijuana plant. While CBD is a component of marijuana (one of hundreds), by itself it does not cause a "high." According to a report from the World Health Organization, "In humans, CBD exhibits no effects indicative of any abuse or dependence potential…. To date, there is no evidence of public health related problems associated with the use of pure CBD."

Is CBD Legal?

CBD is readily obtainable in most parts of the United States, though its exact legal status is in flux. All 50 states have laws legalizing CBD with varying degrees of restriction, and while the federal government still considers CBD in the same class as marijuana, it doesn't habitually enforce against it. In December 2015, the FDA eased the regulatory requirements to allow researchers to conduct CBD trials. Currently, many people obtain CBD online without a medical cannabis license. The **government's position** on CBD is confusing, and depends in part on whether the CBD comes from hemp or marijuana. The legality of CBD has changed, as Congress made the hemp crop legal and for all intents and purposes, makes CBD difficult to prohibit.

CBD has been touted for a wide variety of health issues, but the strongest scientific evidence is for its effectiveness in treating some of the cruelest childhood epilepsy syndromes, such as Dravet syndrome and Lennox-Gastaut syndrome (LGS), which typically don't respond to antiseizure medications. In numerous studies, CBD was able to reduce the number of seizures, and in some cases, it was able to stop them altogether. Videos of the effects of CBD on these children and their seizures are readily available on the Internet for viewing, and they are quite striking. Recently the FDA approved the first ever cannabis-derived medicine for these conditions, Epidiolex, which contains CBD.

CBD is commonly used to address anxiety, and for patients who suffer through the misery of insomnia, studies suggest that CBD may help with both falling asleep and staying asleep.

CBD may offer an option for treating different types of chronic pain. A study from the *European Journal of Pain* showed, using an animal model, CBD applied on the skin could help lower pain and inflammation due to arthritis. Another study demonstrated the mechanism by which CBD inhibits inflammatory and neuropathic pain, two of the most difficult types of chronic pain to treat. More study in humans is needed in this area to substantiate the claims of CBD proponents about pain control.

Is CBD safe?

Side effects of CBD include nausea, fatigue and irritability. CBD can increase the level in your blood of the blood thinner coumadin, and it can raise levels of certain other medications in your blood by the exact same mechanism that grapefruit juice does. A significant safety concern with CBD is that it is primarily marketed and sold as a supplement, not a medication. Currently, the FDA does not regulate the safety and purity of dietary supplements. So, you cannot know for sure that the product you buy has active ingredients at the dose listed on the label. In addition, the product may contain other (unknown) elements.

When purchasing CBD oil, always ask for a Certificate of Analysis (COA) which shows the results of third-party testing performed on the product. The COA will show if the product passed testing for mold and pesticides, as well as, the amount of cannabinoids in the product and the THC level. Several companies have started placing QR codes right on the label enabling you to scan the code with your smartphone in order to link you directly with a website or document with the COA for that particular product. THC-free CBD products have now become available as well, although there is a strong belief among CBD users that products with THC work better. It has been suggested to use THC-free products for day-time use, and to use products with THC at night.

It is also suggested when buying CBD tinctures, to choose "full spectrum" instead of "isolates" due to the term "the entourage effect." The entourage effect is the theory of cannabinoid and terpene synergy. The theory postulates that the use of the **whole plant**, with the hundreds of different chemical compounds, is more medically beneficial than isolated cannabinoids and terpenes. Terpenes cannabinoids and flavonoids all work together to improve their medical benefit, or to counteract certain side effects. Whole plant cannabis products are better than the sum of their individual parts, and a more balanced approach to cannabis as medicine.

We cannot talk about CBD without discussing cannabinoids and terpenes, as well as our body's endocannabinoid system!

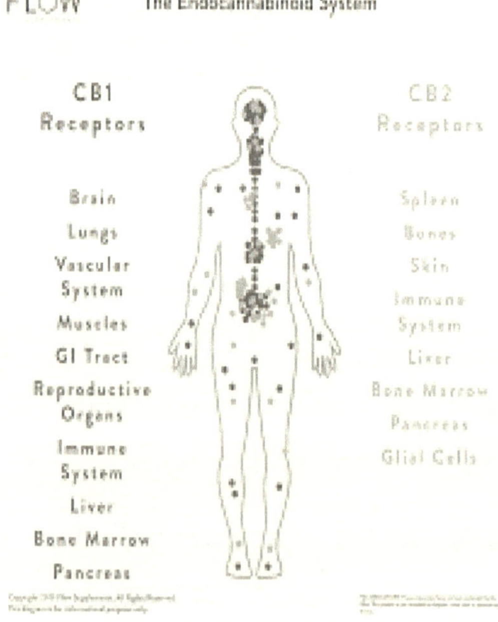

Figure 7 - Endocannabinoid System

Cannabinoids and the Human Body

Cannabinoids are naturally occurring chemical compounds. They are bioactive metabolites. Originally isolated from the cannabis plant in the 1940's, scientists have now uncovered them in many other medicinally beneficial plants including Theobroma cacao (chocolate), echinacea (coneflower), and radula marginata (liverwort).

Cannabis contains more than 113 cannabinoids, producing diverse effects on the human body. In marijuana, cannabinoids are a viscous resin originating from the glands, known as trichomes, of the plant. Along with other chemical compounds, including terpenes and flavonoids, the trichomes protect the flowers from disease, pests, and environmental threats. The phytocannabinoids produced by cannabis, and other plants, interact seamlessly with the human endocannabinoid system. They replicate and improve the characteristics of endocannabinoids. Each cannabinoid has a unique effect on the human body and have powerful medicinal qualities.

MAJOR CANNABINOIDS

	Medicinal Benefit	Effects	Side Effects
Tetrahydrocann abidiol (THC)	Analgesic, anti-inflammatory, anti-tumor, chemotherapy co-treatment to reduce nausea and vomiting, neuroprotectant, sedative, improves appetite, antioxidant, antibacterial	Psychoactive, it's the only cannabinoid responsible for the cerebral 'high' associated with cannabis. Depending on combination with other compounds can be energetic, euphoric, relaxing and/or stress-relieving.	Paranoia, anxiety, increased appetite, short term cognitive impairment, dry mouth
Cannabidiol	Anti-inflammatory, anti-tumor, anti-anxiety, mood regulatory, sleep-aid (low doses), anticonvulsant (anti-seizure), immune modulator	Non-psychoactive, relaxing, mood-regulating, stress relief, mild to no sensation.	Rare and mild changes in appetite, diarrhea, drowsiness

MINOR CANNABINOIDS

	Medicinal Benefit	Effects	Side Effects
(CBG) Cannabigerol	Anti-inflammatory, analgesic, muscle relaxant, immune	Non-psychoactive, relaxing, mood-regulating, stress relief, mild to no	N/A

	modulator, digestive aid, anti-anxiety	sensation	
(CBC) **Cannabichrome ne**	Anti-inflammatory, anti-anxiety, anti-bacterial, analgesic	Non-psychoactive, relaxing, mood regulating, mild to no sensation	N/A
(CBN) **Cannabinol**	Sedative, anti-inflammatory, anti-bacterial, improves appetite	Non-psychoactive, relaxing, mild to no sensation	N/A
(THCV) **Tetrahydrocann abivarin**	Anti-inflammatory, anti-anxiety, appetite suppression, blood sugar regulation, anticonvulsant	Unknown if psychoactive (may be based on dose), stress relief, mild to no sensation	Mild appetite suppression

The endocannabinoid system (ECS) is an extensive system of receptors and chemical communications. All mammals have an ECS, which keeps the body in balance in response to the internal and external stressors. It is the bridge between the body and the mind. Discovered in 1990 by a team of researchers studying cannabis' effect on the human body.

- Receptors located throughout the body mostly concentrated in the brain, glands, organs, connective tissues, central nervous system, and immune cells.

- Regulates mood, memory, learning, pain, appetite, immune system, reproduction, and digestions.

- Humans ECS produces natural endocannabinoids including anandamide, 2-arachidonoylglycerol, and N-Arachidonoyl dopamine.

- In response to stressors (infections, injury, mood fluctuations, stress) the ECS releases neurological transmissions, which travel to the relevant area and work to return the system to homeostatis.

- Interacts seamlessly with phytocannabinoids, including those found in cannabis.

- Two primary endocannabinoid receptors, CB1 and CB2.

CB1 Receptors are primarily concentrated in the brain, central nervous and reproductive systems. It is also thought to regulate cardiovascular function. The primary cannabinoid in cannabis, THC, interacts almost exclusively with this receptor.

CB2 Receptors are primarily concentrated within the immune system. Cannabinoids have less direct relationship with the CB2 receptor, yet still influence its function.

- Cannabinoids either activate or inhibit endocannabinoid receptor activity.

- Cannabinoids can also increase or decrease the effects of human's endocannabinoids.

- Effects can be entirely dose-dependent, with low doses attributed to to one result and high doses triggering an opposite effect.

- Most cannabinoids indirectly interact with CB1 and CB2 receptors and do not form a direct link.

- THC, the only known psychoactive cannabinoid, forms a direct link with the CB1 receptor in the brain. The THC molecule fits like a key into a lock, with the CB1 receptor. The relationship is responsible for the "high."

- Once absorbed by the bloodstream, cannabinoids metabolize into other compounds. These compounds are then stored in fat cells.

- Only THC is psychoactive.

> ➤ Drug testing only tests for THC and the related metabolites. There are no drug tests for other cannabinoids.

Terpenes

There are more than 20,000 terpenes, with more than a hundred in cannabis alone. Terpenes are volatile aromatic oils produced by cannabis as a natural defense against pests and disease. Like cannabinoids, terpenes are a product of the trichome. Many common plants produce the same terpenes also produced by the cannabis plant, including citrus fruits, herbs, and other medicinal plants.

Terpenes are also responsible for the unique flavors and aromas, which define individual strains. They are also responsible in part for nuanced experiences of each strain, including various medicinal benefits. They are similar to cannabinoids in the sense they have different heat sensitivities, effects and medicinal benefits.

TERPENE	AROMA	ALSO FOUND IN	EFFECTS	MEDICINAL BENEFIT
Myrcene	Herbal, musky, cardamom	Mango, lemongrass, thyme	Sedative, relaxing, calming, synergistic	Sleep aid, muscle relaxant, analgesic,

			with THC	anti-inflammatory, anticonvulsant
Limonene	Citrus, lemon	Lemon, lime, peppermint	Energizing, uplifting, stress relief, increases attention	Mood disorders, antifungal, antibacterial, improves immune system, digestive aid
Terpinoline	Herbal, pine, floral	Tea tree, cumin, apples	Sedative, relaxing, stress relief	Antibacterial, antifungal, anti-tumor, sleep aid
Beta-Caryophyllene	Spicy, peppery, cloves	Black pepper, cinnamon, cloves	Unknown	Analgesic, anti-inflammatory, antifungal, neuro protectant, anti-tumor
Pinene	Pine, forest	Conifer trees, rosemary, basil	Energetic, improves memory, and may reduce the effects of THC	Antioxidant, anti-inflammatory, antihistamine, anti-cancer, bronchodilator
Humulene	Earthy, hops, musty	Hops, basil, coriander	Sedative, appetite control, synergistic with terpenes and cannabinoids	Antibacterial, anti-inflammatory, anti-tumor, appetite suppressant, antihistamine
Linalool	Floral	Lavender, mint,	Stress relief, sedative,	Mood disorders,

		rosewood	mood enhancing	(anxiety, depression), sleep-aid, analgesic, anticonvulsant
Ocimene	Sweet, herbal, woodsy	Mint, basil, kumquats	Uplifting, mood enhancer	Anti-inflammatory, antiviral, antifungal, decongestant

Known Synergistic Relationships in Cannabis

THC + CBD

- CBD naturally reduces the length and strength of the 'high' associated with THC by decreasing the period THC locks with the CB1 receptor.

- A small level of THC is required to improve the medicinal qualities of CBD.

- THC has powerful properties useful for chronic pain.

- CBD is a powerful anti-inflammatory, and also though to target neuropathic pain.

THC + THCV

- THCV counteracts the powerful appetite stimulation of THC

THC + Myrcene

- THC is a sleep aid and sedative

- Myrcene may contribute to the 'couch lock' sedative effects of many cannabis strains

CBD + Limonene + Linalool

- CBD promotes a decrease in lipid (fat) production in acne

- Limonene works better than common pharmaceuticals to reduce the signs of acne

- Linalool reduces acne triggered inflammation

- CBD has well established anti-anxiety and anti-depressant qualities

- Limonene and linalool terpenes also both have anti-anxiety and anti-depressant properties

CBD + CBG + Pinene

- CBD and CBG inhibit Methicillin-resistant Staphylococcus aureus (MRSA) growth

- Pinene is equal to or more effective than common pharmaceuticals for the treatment of MRSA

- Pinene improves skin permeability, increasing the effectiveness of other medications.

The bottom line on CBD

Some CBD manufacturers have come under government scrutiny for wild, indefensible claims, such that CBD is a cure-all for cancer, which it is not. We need more research but CBD may be prove to be an option for managing anxiety, insomnia, and chronic pain. Without sufficient high-quality evidence in human studies we can't pinpoint effective doses, and because CBD is currently is mostly available as an unregulated supplement, it's difficult to know exactly what you are getting. If you decide to try CBD, talk with your doctor — if for no other reason than to make sure it won't affect other medications you are taking.

Chapter 5

Dosage

The following calculations work for any listed cannabinoid content, THC is used as an example.

RAW FLOWER

Product potency (%) x total product (mg) = total mg THC

Total mg of THC/number of doses = mg of THC per dose

Example: 1 gram of cannabis rolled into 4 (0.25 g) joints 13% THC product potency x 1000 mg of product = 130 mg of total THC

130 mg total THC/4 joints = 32.5 mg of THC per joint

EDIBLE

Total THC per package/number of servings = mg of THC per dose

Example: 100 mg of THC in a Rice Krispy square

100 mg/10 servings = 10 mg of THC per serving

TINCTURE OR OIL

Total THC per bottle (mg)/Total volume of tincture per bottle (ml) – Total mg per ml

1 dropper full of liquid = 1 ml

1 dropper full = 30 drops

Example: 100 mg of THC in 15 ml bottle

100 mg THC/ 20 ml = 5 mg per ml

1 dropper full = 5 mg

5mg/ 30 drops = 0.016 mg of THC per drop of tincture

Guide to Quantities

GRAM	Size of a single grape
1/8 OUNCE	Size of a Kiwi
¼ OUNCE	Size of an Apple
½ OUNCE	Size of a Grapefruit
1 OUNCE	Size of a Coconut

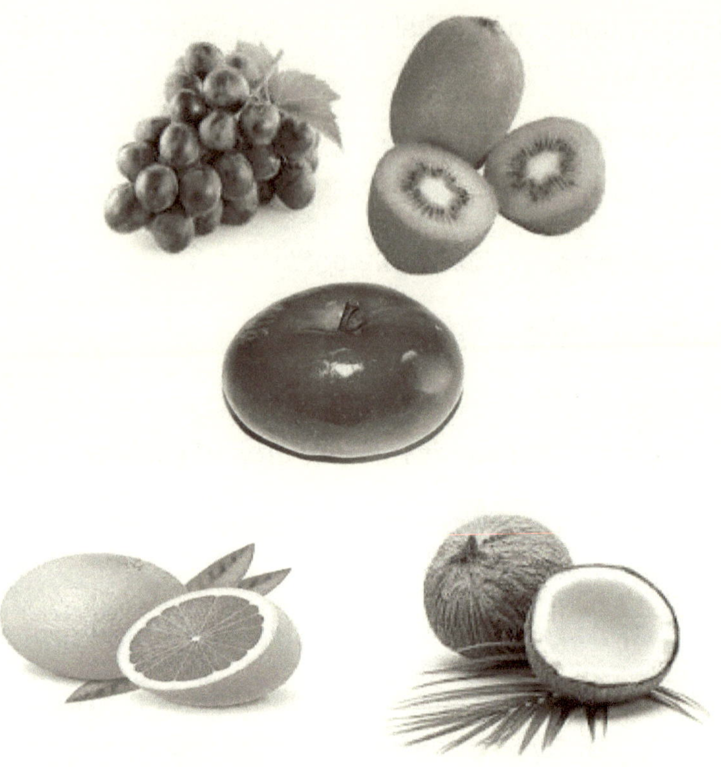

Dosing Ratios and Expected Effects of CBD:THC

CBD	THC	EFFECT
0	1	High potency. With no CBD component, THC delivers a long lasting and strongly psychoactive high. Higher risk of adverse side effects including anxiety and discomfort
1	2	Medium-High potency. Small CBD component mitigates the psychoactive experience and reduces the risk of anxiety and other side effects
1	1	Medium potency. Mild and more comfortable psychoactive effect.

		Less risk of anxiety, typically more euphoric.
2	1	Mild potency. Mild to subtle psychoactive effect, depending on the tolerance of the individual.
1	0	No potency. No psychoactive effects, and no risk of adverse reaction causing anxiety.

Suggested Dosing Tables for CBD Tinctures

LOW POTENCY OR <u>CBD ONLY</u> SUGGESTED SELF TITRATION SCHEDULE

DAY	MORNING	EVENING
Day 1-3	0 Drops	10 Drops
Day 4-6	0 Drops	30 Drops
Day 7-9	8 Drops	30 Drops
Day 10-12	10 Drops	20 Drops

Day 13-15	15 Drops	25 Drops
Day 16-18	20 Drops	30 Drops
Day 19-21	30 Drops	30 Drops

MEDIUM POTENCY OR 1:1 THC to CBD SUGGESTED SELF TITRATION SCHEDULE

DAY	MORNING	EVENING
Day 1-3	0 Drops	8 Drops
Day 4-6	8 Drops	8 Drops
Day 7-9	8 Drops	15 Drops
Day 10-12	15 Drops	15 Drops
Day 13-15	15 Drops	20 Drops
Day 16-18	20 Drops	20 Drops
Day 19-21	20 Drops	30 Drops

HIGH POTENCY OR THC ONLY SUGGESTED SELF TITRATION SCHEDULE

DAY	MORNING	EVENING
Day 1-3	0 Drops	2 Drops
Day 4-6	0 Drops	4 Drops
Day 7-9	0 Drops	15 Drops
Day 10-12	0 Drops	20 Drops
Day 13-15	0 Drops	30 Drops

HOW TO MICRO-DOSE

GOAL: To avoid adverse reaction and psychoactive effects of THC. Therapeutic benefit without the high.

SUGGESTED PRODUCTS: Cannabis tinctures with dose dropper, vaporizer with dose control, one-hitter pipe with raw flower, and capsules with pre-measured doses of concentrate.

DOSING GUIDELINES:

√ Start with 1-2 mg per dose.

√ Increase only if no side effects are experienced.

√ Maximum dose under 10 mg per serving.

√ Patients may micro-dose multiple times per day to achieve therapeutic benefit but must avoid cognitive impairment, euphoria and paranoia.

CHAPTER 6

CBD for Pets

CBD is a popular home remedy and an alternative natural prescription provided by some veterinarians. CBD has a high safety profile for humans, cats, dogs, and other mammals. It is safe for day and night-time use, for a variety of health conditions, and ages. Under the guidance of a veterinarian, it is also safe to use in conjunction with other medications.

MEDICAL BENEFITS

Arthritis and Inflammation

- Dogs respond well to CBD for arthritis related pain and inflammation.

- CBD is a well-established anti-inflammatory agent in preliminary studies on human health conditions.

- Studies on dogs with osteoarthritis recorded no measurable side effects, increased comfort and increased activity.

- The study used a dose of 2mg/kg delivered two times daily.

- Applications: The treatment of arthritis, osteoarthritis, stiff muscles and joints, and mobility issues.

Pain

- CBD reduces inflammatory and neuropathic pain models.

- Studies on dogs with inflammatory diseases recorded positive effects on pain and comfort levels.

- The compound has a higher safety profile than comparable prescribed medicines and no tolerance development.

- Applications: The treatment of pain related to injury, age arthritis, and inflammation.

Anxiety and Aggression

- Aggression and agitation in dogs are often tied to stress and anxiety.

- In human studies, CBD is a proven anti-anxiety compound, through its ability to boost serotonin receptor signaling.

- CBD helps reduce nervousness by improving endocannabinoid signaling.

- Applications: The treatment of excess agitation, separation anxiety, anxiety-related aggression, anxiety related to neglect and abuse, and anxiety related to loud noise (fireworks).

Seizures

- Certain dog breeds are susceptible to genetically triggered seizures, shown to decrease in severity and frequency when treated with CBD.

- In humans, CBD is an approved pharmaceutical for intractable forms of childhood epilepsy.

- Studies on lab rats with epilepsy showed CBD was more effective for treating seizures than Phenytoin and Ethosuximide.

- Applications: The treatment of dog and cat forms of epilepsy, with or without co-treatment and conventional medications.

Cancer

- Preliminary evidence suggests cannabinoids, including CBD, target cancerous cells.

- May reduce metastasis, promote cell apoptosis, and reduce tumor size of certain cancers.

- Applications: A natural therapy useful for combination with other conventional cancer treatments.

Palliative Care

- Animals often suffer from muscle and joint pain, loss of appetite, lethargy, inflammation and more as they age.

- CBD reduces inflammation, increases appetite and improves quality of life during the final stages.

- Applications: To provide comfort and increase quality of life during palliative care.

Safety and Precautions

- THC is not suitable for therapeutic applications with pets.

- THC interacts with the CB1 endocannabinoid receptors in the mammalian brain.

- Animals have more cannabinoid receptors in their brains than humans, making THC poisonous to other animals – including dogs and cats.

- Humans generally respond to positively to THC: a high, euphoria, and temporary cognitive impairment.

- THC quickly overwhelmed the non-human brain leading to an unpleasant, dangerous and possibly lethal experience.

- Dogs are at higher risk for consumption of non-pet cannabis products, especially cannabis-infused edibles including chocolates.

- Chocolates and other common edible ingredients are also harmful to dogs, triggering multiple toxicities.

- Smaller dogs are more susceptible to dangerous overdoses due to their small size.

- Cats rarely consume cannabis edibles, although may ingest raw flower.

- Cats also have a strong negative reaction to THC.

SIGNS OF PET POISONING

- Difficulties with motor function

- Problems with balance

- Dizziness

- Abnormal or slow responses

- Incontinence

- Agitation

- Sedation

- Increased or decreased heart rate

- Vomiting

▶ IN CASE OF EMERGENCY ◀

- Contact emergency veterinarian services immediately!

- Keep water available!

- Do not try to induce vomiting!

- Recovery may take upwards of 24 hours!

- May require overnight monitoring or a stomach pump!

Types of CBD Products for Pets

PRODUCT	INFO	HOW TO USE
Treats (Pet Edibles)	The most common CBD pet product is a CBD-infused pet edible combined with conventional pet-suitable foods, like proteins, grains and vegetables. They are easy to deliver and usually well received. Some edibles include other medicinal ingredients.	Read the package for instructions before use and daily recommendation.
Oils and Tinctures	The second most common CBD pet product is an oil or tincture.	Using the dropper, dose oil over the top of wet or dry

	CBD is suspended within a pet-friendly carrier oil such as coconut, olive oil or MCT oil. Potencies may vary, read the label for CBD concentration and dosing guidelines.	food or directly into the pat's mouth. Read the package for instructions before use. Calculate daily CBD dose based on weight and product potency.
Capsules	Useful for higher doses. Although may be challenging to deliver for some pill-adverse pets. Capsules are usually vegetable-based, with higher potency than other products.	If the pet is not receptive to pills, capsules may be hidden inside pill pockets or wet food for easy delivery. Read the package for instructions before use. Calculate daily CBD dose based on weight and product potency.
Topicals	Often combined with other medicinal	Easy to use and apply to the area of concern.

	ingredients, CBD infused topicals provide relief for sore muscles, inflamed joints, and minor skin irritations. Some CBD pet products are designed to relieve dry, irritated and sore paw pads. Safe if accidentally ingested.	CBD does not penetrate the skin, and there are no restrictions on dose.

Dosage and Titration Using CBD Oil for Pets

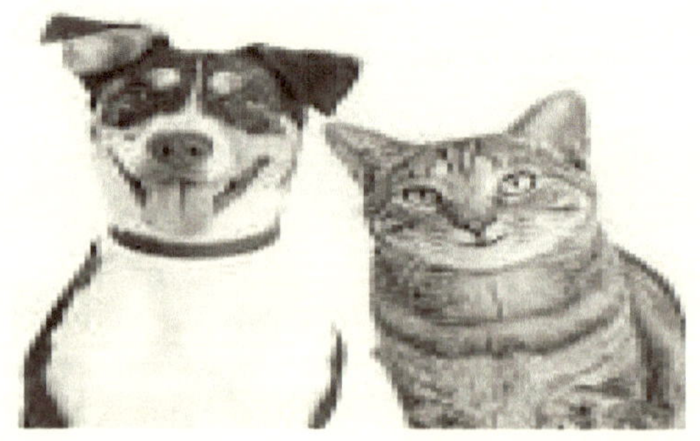

Figure 8 - Dog and Cat

Always review product label for specific product dosing instructions. If prescribed by a veterinarian, follow dosing instructions! Follow standard dosage calculation in all other cases, which requires input on: pet weight (lbs), the concentration of CBD per ml of tincture/oil, and the severity of the medical condition, disease or illness (low, middle or high).

Daily Dosage Chart for Dogs

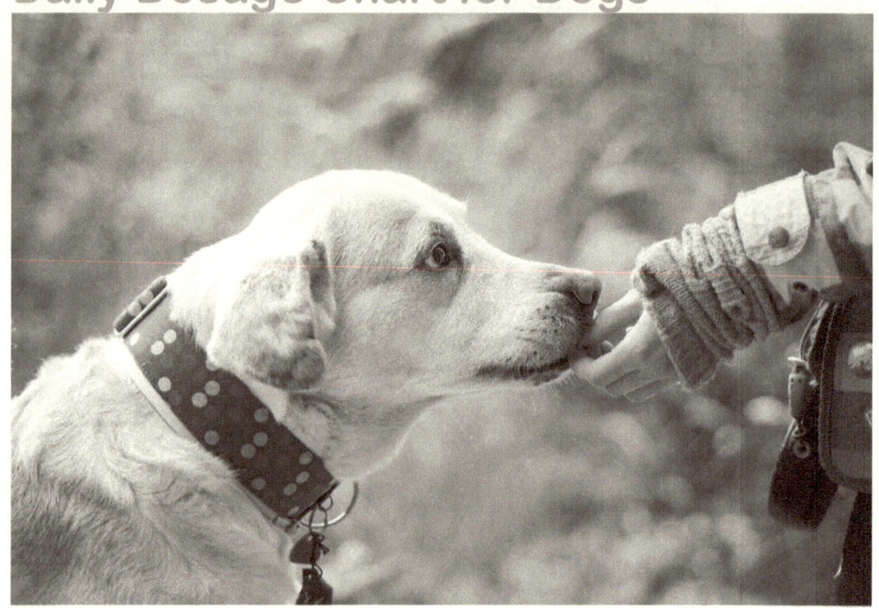

Figure 9 – Dog

Weight (lbs)	Low (mg)	Middle (mg)	High (mg)
Two Doses Daily – Morning and Evening			
2	0.10	0.25	0.50
5	0.25	0.65	1.25
10	0.50	1.25	2.50
15	0.75	1.85	3.75
20	1.00	2.50	5.00

25	1.25	3.15	6.25
Weight (lbs)	Low (mg)	Middle (mg)	High (mg) *cont.*
30	1.50	3.75	7.50
35	1.75	4.35	8.75
40	2.00	5.00	10.00
45	2.25	5.65	11.25
50	2.50	6.25	12.50
60	3.00	7.50	15.00
70	3.50	8.75	17.50
80	4.00	10.00	20.00
90	4.50	11.25	22.50
100	5.00	12.50	25.00

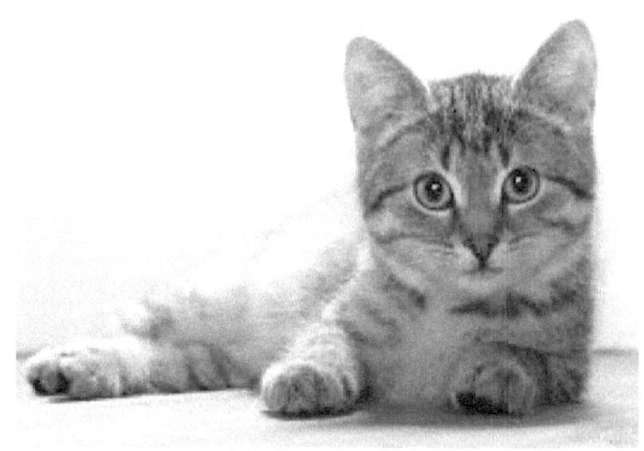

Daily Dosage Chart for Cats

Weight (lbs)	Low (mg)	Middle (mg)	High (mg)

Two Doses Daily – Morning and Evening

2	0.10	0.25	0.50
5	0.25	0.65	1.25
10	0.50	1.25	2.50
15	0.75	1.85	3.75
20	1.00	2.50	5.00

CBD Pet Edible Recipes

CBD Coconut Oil Treats and Topical

- 2 cups coconut oil
- 30 ml CBD Tincture

1. Calculate or record total CBD in mg from the tincture label

2. Slowly melt coconut oil in a saucepan over low heat

3. Remove from heat and allow to cool for 10 minutes.

4. While still a liquid, combine with CBD tincture. Stir well.

5. Depending on the preferred method of delivery, pour into a plastic container or silicone chocolate mold. Place in freezer to harden for 4 hours.

6. Recalculate potency of CBD per ml of the coconut oil mixture.

7. Label container with dose, and store in the freezer up to 6 months.

To use: Coconut oil infused can be given to dogs as-is, melted and combined with daily meals, spread inside a chew toy, or used topically.

Frozen Pumpkin CBD Dog Treats

- 1 cup pure pumpkin puree
- ½ cup plain Greek yogurt
- 20-30 ml CBD tincture

1. Calculate or record total CBD in mg from the tincture label.

2. Combine all ingredients into a large mixing bowl.

3. Mix well and combine.

4. Pour mixture into an ice cream tray, or silicone mold and freeze.

5. Recalculate CBD dose per serving of pumpkin oil mixture.

6. Label container with dose, and store in the freezer for up to 3 months,

To use: Individual sections can be given with meals or as a treat. Especially useful if capsules or tinctures are not well received by the pet.

CBD Dog Bones

- 2/3 cup apple sauce
- ¼ cup peanut butter
- 2 large eggs
- ¼ cup coconut oil
- 3 cups high-quality flour
- 1 tsp baking soda
- 30 ml CBD tincture

1. Preheat oven to 350 degrees.

2. Combine all ingredients into large bowl, except flour.

3. Slowly add flour in small batches while stirring. Eventually, begin to knead dough until well formed.

4. Roll out dough into 1/3 inch to ½ inch thickness. Use a bone shaped cookie dough cutter to cut forms.

5. Line cookie sheet with parchment paper, and place cookies on the sheet.

6. Bake for 15 minutes and allow to cool before storage.

7. Recalculate dosage per cookie (30 ml / X of cookies)

8. Label dose and date on the container. Store in airtight container at room temperature for up to 1 week or in the refrigerator for 2 weeks.

CHAPTER 7

Cooking with Cannabis

A cannabis edible is a foodstuff infused with cannabinoids and terpenes from marijuana. Common infusions include cooking oils and fats such as olive oil, butter, or coconut oil. Alcohol-based tinctures, solvent-based cannabis extractions, and isolates are also edible. Infusing cannabis into foods has a long history of use. A sweet, creamy preparation called Bhang, a beverage used historically within Hindu religious ceremonies, dates back to at least 1000 B.C. In Western medicine, cannabis tinctures rose in popularity during the 1800's for the treatment of convulsions, inflammation and childbirth. The counter-culture of the 1960's used cannabis edibles as a recreational past time, developing a reputation for infused brownies and space cakes. With the rise of legal recreational cannabis post-2000, commercial edible production began on a large scale. Cannabis edibles come in a variety of formats including pastries, candies, cakes, teas, beverages, savory dishes, sauces and more.

BENEFITS OF COOKING WITH CANNABIS

- Medicinally provides long-term, powerful relief of chronic issues like pain, inflammation, palliative needs, and cancer.

- Recreationally stimulates a deeper, more relaxing psychoactive experience than inhaled methods.

- Slow release of medicinal or recreational compounds, lasting 6 to 10 hours.

- Useful for the consumption of high doses.

- Edibles stimulate higher sensations of sedation, compared to other methods of ingestion (smoking, vaping).

- Avoids the development of respiratory health issues associated with inhaled cannabis.

- Cannabis infusions are highly adaptable: sweet to savory; Indian to French; breakfast to dinner.

BASICS OF CANNABIS EDIBLES

Format: Onset: slow, 30 to 60 minutes.

Duration: Long term, 6 to 10 hours.

Risk: Acute, marijuana intoxication is mot commonly triggered by an edible, due to the comparably inaccurate mechanism of dosing and the lengthy onset of relief.

HOW TO DOSE EDIBLES

- Standard single serving: 10 mg of THC.

- Commercial edibles often come in packages containing multiple doses.

- Dose only one serving (10 mg) to start.

- More experienced users can start with higher doses, proceed with caution.

- Wait at least 2 hours after the initial dose, before consuming more.

Cooking with Cannabis Dose Calculation

CALCULATING THC

(Total product in mg) x (potency %) = (THC content in mg)

Example: 10,000 mg x 10% THC = 1000 mg of THC

CALCULATE THC PER CUP OF FAT/OIL

(THC content in mg) / (Fat/Oil in cups) = (THC content per cup)

Example: 1000 mg of THC / 4 cups butter = 250 mg of THC per cup of butter

CALCULATE THC PER SERVING

(THC content per cup) x (number of cups used) = (Total THC per dish)

Example: 250 mg THC x 2 cups butter in the recipe = 500 mg THC in the final dish

(Total THC per dish) / (number of servings) = (THC potency per serving)

Example: 500 mg / 25 servings = 25 mg of THC per serving

Acute Marijuana Intoxication

Edibles are the leading cause of acute marijuana intoxication. The effects of acute marijuana intoxication are alarming and uncomfortable but are non-life threatening.

INITIAL SYMPTOMS: Euphoria, Time and spatial distortion, intensification of sensory experiences, cognitive impairment and motor impairment.

ACUTE SYMPTOMS: Low blood pressure, panic, short-term psychotic, anxiety, involuntary muscle jerking, delirium, respiratory depression, lack of muscle coordination.

HOW TO REDUCE THE RISK OF ACUTE MARIJUANA INTOXICATION

- If sensitive to THC, introduce slowly in micro-doses (under 5 mg)

- Introduce THC before going to sleep at night, before ingesting during the day.

- Combine with equal doses of CBD to reduce psychoactive experience.

- Never consume an edible without knowing the dose.

- Never consume a second dose within 2 hours of the first dose.

- To prevent accidental intoxication, clearly label all edibles as food which contain THC.

- Keep all edibles out of the reach of children!

TREATMENT OF ACUTE MARIJUANA INTOXICATION

- Intoxication is typically short term, lasting for 24 hours or less and the most challenging symptoms lasting for under 6.

- Treatment of acute intoxication is exclusively about symptom management including:

  - Deep breathing

  - Comfort from a close friend or family member

  - Drinking water

  - Sleep

- Seek medical assistance for accidental consumption involving children or seniors with no experience with cannabis.

- Seek medical assistance for those who have entered into psychosis.

The Decarboxylation Process (Decarbing)

Decarboxylation is a molecular change following exposure to heat over time. Decarbing is the first step to cooking with cannabis. It is crucial to transforming many of the chemical compounds in cannabis into medicinally and recreationally active compounds.

Raw cannabis flower contains cannabinoids in the acid formation including: THCA, CBDA, and CBGA. Cannabis, after exposure to heat over time, transforms acidic cannabinoids into activated ones by removing the carboxyl group. Examples include: THCA into THC, CBDA into CBD, CBGA into CBG, and THCA into CBN.

Smoking, vaping and baking are effective ways to decarb cannabis into activated compounds before cooking with cannabis, it is essential to decarb the raw plant material to trigger this shift.

HOW TO DECARB CANNABIS

1. Set oven to 240 degrees (115 degrees Celsius)

2. Roughly grind the cannabis flower.

3. Line a cookie sheet with parchment paper and spread ground flower in an even layer on the tray.

4. Cover with tinfoil.

5. Place the tray in the oven for between 45 to 60 minutes. Different strains with cannabinoid combinations, decarboxylate at varying rates. Do not decarb for more than 60 minutes to avoid THC loss.

6. Remove foil and allow to cool.

7. Store in a sealed container in a cool, dry place until ready to use. Do not refrigerate.

INCORPORATING FATS INTO INFUSIONS

- Cannabinoids (THC and CBD) are lipophiles (fat-soluble) and hydrophobic (water-adverse) compounds.

- Consuming cannabis with fat improves their bioavailability (absorption rate).

- Cannabinoids inhaled by smoking and vaping, absorb directly through the respiratory track.

- Ingested cannabinoids must absorb through the digestive track and require fats to do so effectively.

- The body metabolizes cannabinoids through the liver and stores the cannabinoid metabolites in fat cells around the body.

- Cannabis edibles without fats still contain medicinal and recreational value, but the benefits increase with the addition of fat.

- Common fats for cannabis infusions include cooking oils like olive oil and avocado oil, dairy products like butter and milk, and vegan options like coconut butter.

Cannabis Recipes

CANNABIS OIL INFUSION (VEGAN)

Uses:

- Vegan alternative

- Substitute for cooking oil in baking (brownies, cake mixes)

- Substitute for cooking oil in savory dishes (Italian dishes, sauces, BBQ)

- Do not fry with infused oil!

•

INGREDIENTS

½ ounce cannabis

1 cup cooking oil (olive oil, avocado, or other suitable oil)

1 tsp sunflower lecithin (emulsifier)

1. Decarboxylate the cannabis before using. Spread the cannabis on an oven tray, covered with foil or parchment. Cover with tin foil.

2. Bake for 45 minutes at 240 degrees F. Allow to cool.

3. Roughly grind the cannabis to the consistency of dried culinary herbs.

4. Add cannabis, cooking oil, and emulsifier into large mason jar.

5. Place the jar with cover on in cold water and let it come to a simmer.

6. Simmer for 3 hours.

7. Remove from heat and allow to cool.

8. Strain through a cheesecloth.

9. Store in a glass container in a cool, dark place for 1 to 2 weeks at room temperature, or up to 6 weeks in the refrigerator.

CANNABIS COCONUT OIL INFUSION (VEGAN)

Uses:

- Vegan alternative

- Healthy fat

- Substitute for coconut oil in savory dishes (curries, stir fry)

- Use topically as a massage oil

- Do not fry with infused coconut oil!

INGREDIENTS:

½ ounce cannabis

1 cup coconut oil (refined, unrefined)

1 tsp sunflower lecithin (emulsifier)

1. Decarboxylate the cannabis before using. (see previous recipes)

2. Bake for 45 minutes at 240 degrees F.

3. Roughly grind the cannabis to the consistency of dried culinary herbs.

4. Add cannabis, coconut oil, and emulsifier into a large

mason jar.

5. Place the jar with cover on in cold water and let it come to a simmer.

6. Simmer for 3 hours.

7. Remove from heat and allow to cool.

8. Strain through a cheesecloth.

9. Store in a sealed container in refrigerator or freezer. Good for 1 – 2 weeks at room temperature or 6 weeks in refrigerator.

CANNABIS BUTTER INFUSION (DAIRY)

Uses:

- Healthy fat

- Substitute for butter in baking

- Substitute for butter in savory dishes

- Substitute for butter spread

- Do not fry with infused butter!

INGREDIENTS:

½ ounce cannabis

1 cup butter

1 tsp sunflower lecithin

1. Decarboxylate the cannabis before using. (see previous recipes)

2. Roughly grind the cannabis to the consistency of dried culinary herbs.

3. Add cannabis, coconut oil, and emulsifier into a large mason jar.

4. Place the jar with cover on in cold water and let it come to a simmer.

5. Simmer for 3 hours.

6. Remove from heat and allow to cool.

7. Strain through a cheesecloth.

8. Store in a sealed container, in refrigerator or freezer for 6 weeks in the refrigerator or 6 months in the freezer.

CANNABIS SUGAR

Uses:

Stirred into a hot beverage (coffee, hot chocolate, tea) and used in baking (cookies, treats, candies)

INGREDIENTS:

¼ cup cannabis tincture

2 cups sugar

1. Add all ingredients in a mixing bowl and mix well.

2. Spread sugar mixture over a cookie sheet lined with parchment paper.

3. Allow to dry exposed for 12 hours.

4. Break off chunks of sugar and break up in a blender until normal sugar consistency is achieved.

Store indefinitely although THC potency may deteriorate over time.

NATURAL CANNABIS GUMMY BEARS

Uses:

Precise and accurate dosing, including as a micro-dose.
Portable, easy and discreet method of dosing.

INGREDIENTS:

1 tbsp cannabis tincture

1 cup berries (strawberries, raspberries, etc.)

½ cup water

1 tbsp lemon juice

2 tbsp honey

1/3 oz. gelatin

4 tbsp citric acid

4 tbsp fine sugar

1. Combine berries with water in a blender until smooth.

2. Strain through a sieve into a pot to remove inconsistencies and seeds.

3. Simmer over low heat for 5 minutes.

4. Remove from heat and immediately combine lemon juice and honey.

5. While still warm, add cannabis tincture and gelatin. Stir until dissolved.

6. Divide the mixture into a gummy bear silicone candy mold.

7. Freeze for at least 1 hour until gelatin sets.

8. Combine sugar and citric acid in a small bowl.

9. Remove gummy bears from the mold and toss in sugar mixture.

10. Place in an air-tight container and store for up to 7 days in the refrigerator or up to 1 month in the freezer.

Cannabis Gummy Bears (cont.)

BHANG, A TRADITIONAL HINDU DRINK

Uses:

Gentle infusion for evening use. A classic preparation.

INGREDIENTS:

2 cups water

8 grams cannabis

3 cups milk

½ cup cane sugar

1 tbsp coconut oil

1 tbsp ground almonds

½ tsp ground ginger

A pinch or garam masala

1 tsp grenadine

1. Decarboxylate the cannabis before use. (see previous recipes)

2. Bring water to a boil and combine the cannabis flower.

3. Simmer for 10 minutes over low heat.

4. Remove from heat and strain the mixture to remove cannabis plant matter and transfer to a bowl.

5. Add a few tablespoons milk and ground almonds, stirring continuously.

6. Slowly incorporate all remaining milk, stirring continuously.

7. Add the remaining ingredients and stir to combine.

8. Pour into a serving jug and allow to cool in the refrigerator before serving. Store for 2-3 days in the refrigerator.

Rick Simpson Oil (Medicinal Cannabis Oil)

CAUTION – This technique produces a highly potent extraction with a flammable solvent. The vapors may be toxic with acute exposure. Avoid open flames, stovetops, and sparks. Make this extraction outdoors, or in a well-ventilated area.

Uses: Extremely potent medicinal product, easy and discreet dose, combine into warm dishes (sauces, curries, etc.), combine into hot beverages (coffee, tea)

INGREDIENTS:

1 oz. cannabis

17 oz. high proof grain alcohol (Everclear)

TOOLS:

2 large food-safe plastic buckets

Scissors

Large spoon for stirring

Coffee filter or cheesecloth

Rice cooker or crockpot

Thermometer

Food dehydrator

Plastic syringe

1. Roughly chop cannabis into the plastic bucket, with a pair of scissors.

2. Add ½ of the solvent into the bucket and mix well with the spoon for 3 minutes.

3. Strain the cannabis mixture into a new bucket.

4. Repeat steps 1-3 for the second wash. Add the remaining solvent to the plant material and stir for 3 minutes.

5. Strain the new cannabis-solvent mixture into the bucket containing the first mixture.

6. Discard the plant material.

7. Pour the dark green solvent through a coffee filter into a rice cooker or crockpot (roughly 75 percent full, do not overfill).

8. Set the rice cooker (or crockpot) to high.

9. Monitor the solution with a food safe thermometer, it should never go above 290 degrees F.

10. Continue to add solvent to cooker as it evaporates until there is no solvent mixture remaining.

11. When the solution has reduced to roughly 10-15% of the original mixture, pick up the cooker to gently swirl the mixture around.

12. Reduce the cooking temperature to low setting and continue to swirl every 5 minutes until the solvent has

reduced another 50 percent.

13. Pour into a stainless steel tray and put into a food dehydrator or fruit leather setting for 3-4 hours, until it has achieved the consistency of molasses.

14. Using the plastic syringe, soak up the cannabis oil, or carefully spoon in a sealed container.

15. Store in a cool dry place for 1-2 months at room temperature or for 6 months in the refrigerator.

Rick Simpson Oil (cont.)

Resources

Helpful web links for more information.

MJBiz.com

Ushempauthority.org

Hempsupporter.com

Cannabizdaily.com

Cannabisreports.org

https://www.usda.gov

https://nifa.usda.gov

https://www.ams.usda.gov

Hemp Farming Act of 2018

About the Author

Deana Jones is the founder of Springville Sun Organics CBD, established in 2019. Extensive research went into creating the Springville Sun Organics product line to make sure legality, product safety, and purity regulations were adhered to as well as third party testing, and proper FDA labeling. The idea to establish a CBD product line came from Deana using her knowledge of aromatherapy and alternative natural healing remedies to create a CBD pain balm, and to this day Deana makes each of her popular and effective pain balms by hand. Springville Sun Organics CBD products are available on Facebook under the same name.

Before entering the CBD business, Deana Jones worked in the legal field as a paralegal for 25 years. The importance of research and keeping up with the law on a particular subject cannot be stressed enough and legal veterans view this practice just as important as eating and sleeping! One can never know enough about a subject because the world is always changing.

Deana Jones is known as "Mimi" to her eleven grandchildren, with one more on the way . . . a girl <3

www.ingramcontent.com/pod-product-compliance
Lightning Source LLC
Chambersburg PA
CBHW051212250726
48655CB00006B/2360